Here's to living
Happy First in All
of our circumstances!

# HAPPY FIRST

**HOW TO WIN LIFE IN THE MOMENT
at Home, at Work, at the Gym,
and Even in the kitchen**

# MAUREEN GIBBONS, MD

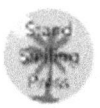

Copyright © 2021 by Maureen Gibbons, M.D.

Cover Design: Cutting-Edge-Studio.com
Typesetting & Formatting: Black Bee Media
Editing: Kim Ledgerwood at TheRightWord.com
Published in the United States by Stand Smiling Press.

All rights reserved.

No part of this publication may be reproduced, distributed, or transmitted in any form or by any means, including photocopying, recording, or other electronic or mechanical methods, without the prior written permission of the publisher, except in the case of brief quotations embodied in critical reviews and certain other noncommercial uses permitted by copyright law.

Although the author and publisher have made every effort to ensure that the information in this book was correct at press time, the author and publisher do not assume and hereby disclaim any liability to any party for any loss, damage, or disruption caused by errors or omissions, whether such errors or omissions result from negligence, accident, or any other cause.

Adherence to all applicable laws and regulations, including international, federal, state, and local governing professional licensing, business practices, advertising, and all other aspects of doing business in the United States, Canada or any other jurisdiction is the sole responsibility of the reader and consumer.

Neither the author nor the publisher assumes any responsibility or liability whatsoever on behalf of the consumer or reader of this material. Any perceived slight of any individual or organization is purely unintentional.

The resources in this book are provided for informational purposes only and should not be used to replace the specialized training and professional judgment of a health care or mental health care professional.

Neither the author nor the publisher can be held responsible for the use of the information provided within this book. Please always consult a trained professional before making any decision regarding treatment of yourself or others.

ISBN: 978-1-7361120-0-7 (Paperback)
ISBN: 978-1-7361120-1-4 (E-Book)

# Dedication

*This book is dedicated to Greg and Matthew.*

*Their support and understanding of my growth and writing made this work possible.*

*In the midst of winter, I found there was,
within me,
an invincible summer.*

~ Albert Camus

# Table of Contents

Dedication .................................................................... *iii*
My Wish for You ............................................... *vii*
Introduction ......................................................... *1*

### Part 1

Chapter 1—What Are You Made Of?................ *5*
Chapter 2—Just a Bit of Weather ...................... *13*
Chapter 3—Abundance....................................... *19*
Chapter 4—Monsters Under the Bed ............... *25*
Chapter 5—Limitless Growth ............................ *31*

### Part 2

Chapter 6—Sleep and Relaxation ..................... *39*
Chapter 7—Nutrition .......................................... *45*
Chapter 8—Activity ............................................ *53*
Chapter 9—Relationships .................................. *59*
Chapter 10—Puppies, Cats, and Caps Lock..... *63*
Chapter 11—Play ................................................. *69*
Chapter 12—The Job Dilemma ......................... *75*
Chapter 13—Time in the Day............................ *79*
Chapter 14—Kindness........................................ *85*
Chapter 15—Conversations............................... *89*

## Part 3

Chapter 16 — Change the Program ..................................97
Chapter 17 — Admiration .................................................103
Chapter 18 — Path of Least Resistance ............................109
Chapter 19 — Doubt Is Inevitable ....................................113
Chapter 20 — Fear Is Expected .........................................115
Chapter 21 — No Need to Bounce....................................119
Chapter 22 — Keep the Channel Open............................121
Chapter 23 — Simple Practices .........................................125
Chapter 24 — Nowhere to Go ...........................................129

Acknowledgments ............................................................133

# My Wish for You

My amazing writing coach told me, "Write the book you're meant to write, not the one you think others want to read. Not everyone will love your book." There are useful tips for everyone in here. Take what you like and leave the rest.

# Introduction

What if you're already happy, but you just don't know it yet?

What if you just need to return to you—the *real* you.

Becoming and living "Happy First" doesn't mean you have to become anyone else; you don't even have to change. The happiness you seek is already inside you. It is your birthright; it is your nature.

Do you feel stressed out? Do you feel like it's too late? Do you feel too fat or too thin? Do you feel too anxious or too apathetic? None of those things are *you*. Most of us don't understand that our joy comes from inside. We look to the outside to provide us with what we believe will make us happy. We get a "better" job, we get a "better" house, a "better" car, a "better" spouse, a "better" body—except nothing makes us feel the way we think it will. So then we try to get more. But it's never enough.

How, then, do we reconnect with that deeper sense of self, the energy inside? There are hundreds of ways to see the real you, in both the easy moments and the uncomfortable ones. It's the latter that are your challenge. When life throws you a curveball—maybe you get a bit of unexpected news or an unpleasant phone call—that's when you get to see your happy shine. Happy First is that bright layer of emotion and energy flowing through it all. Your happiness is straightforward. It is the underlying perfect nature of the universe.

Happy is easier than you think.

# Part 1

# Chapter 1

# What Are You Made Of?

Neither scientists nor clergy can deny the fact that there's an energy that underlies everything that is. Religion calls this God; science may simply call it "energy" and break it down into protons and electrons orbiting about one another. Further still into science, quantum theory has broken open enough of those principles to introduce concepts such as the God particle. Basic scientific education begins to explore the laws of the universe. As far back as 1789, Antoine Lavoisier discovered that matter can neither be created nor destroyed in chemical reactions—also known as the law of conservation of mass. Knowing this, the intellectual leap that your human form has been created solely of energy is not much of a jump at all. The fact that we are created from the same energy that makes up the sun and the trees and what some religions call God isn't a stretch either.

As we learn that energy can neither be created nor destroyed, we can see that energy is often defined by our human brains as light. There is no positive or negative light. There is only light and the absence of it. Some references call that energy "love." If we go by the same principle as the properties of light and love, there can then be no hate. There is only the absence of love. It may change form, but it can neither be created nor destroyed. Life is in flux. Living in an infinite universe, we are reminded that there is no need to "create" love or light. No matter the amount we feel we need, that amount is already present in potential.

Another universal law is that disorder, or entropy, always increases in a closed system. The universe, however, is an open system; it is infinite. The transfer of energy isn't perfect, and some scatters to the surrounding environment. This scientific premise becomes essential when we talk about taking the path of least resistance, also known in this book as "growing toward the sun." Your happiness scatters and "infects" others!

I consider "happiness" to be the expression of that infinite, ever-present energy that creates our reality. Happy First is the concept elucidating how that underlying, immutable, positive energy relates to you and your world. You are made up of light and love and goodness. The expression of this knowledge is the path to living Happy First.

What I do not consider happiness is the solitary pursuit and attainment of external objects and accolades. Michael Neill notes that there is nothing wrong with wanting both peace of mind and a nice piece of real estate.[1]

The two are not mutually exclusive, but it is possible to have wealth without happiness. We see the manifestation of the mindset that conflates wealth with happiness all the time. "If I'm wealthy, I'll be happy." I'm asking you to shake that sentence up. "I'm already happy, but wouldn't it be fun to have a big bank account?" Can you feel the difference between those two sentences? You haven't changed, but your verbal expression of your true nature has.

---

1  Neill, Michael, You Can Have What You Want: Proven Strategies for Inner and Outer Success, (Carlsbad, CA: Hay House, 2006), 6.

being in the water, on my bike, outside running, or even indoors. Each one of these enhances my life differently. Swimming brings me back to when I was supported and encouraged and a very close-knit part of a team. I love biking because I can move fast on my bike, and I'm not a fast person by nature. Running inspires gratitude in me for being able to move on my own two feet.

To give you a bit of background on that, I was a runner before I was a triathlete, and I was inspired to become a runner by a very poignant event. My grandpa was dying, and some family and I were staying at my grandparents' condo about a quarter-mile away from the hospital. We got the call that he was in his last moments, and my dad and I ran to the hospital. We were able to make it in time because we were able-bodied, and we ran. I was grateful to be able to say goodbye. After that, I began to run. I'd never liked to run before because I'm not naturally fast, and I felt a lot of shame around that when I was younger. After my grandfather's passing, my goal was to learn to love the run.

I started out running on a treadmill (it was in Ohio and it was cold) for one minute and walking 29 minutes, three days a week before my medical school clinical duties for the day. The next week, it was two minutes of running and 28 minutes of walking, and so on. Then a friend asked me if I wanted to run a marathon. That seemed incredibly daunting for a non-athletic kid like me. But I thought, "I can do hard things" and told her yes. My first 10K with her was called the Run Happy 10K. Remembering that race and understanding the importance of that race's title brings a huge smile to my face. Run happy, live happy — it's all the same thing. Some days running hard makes you smile; some days running for a minute and walking the rest of the mile makes you smile. But understanding what makes you tick and working *with* yourself instead of against yourself creates an environment of success. Victory as we define it brings us joy.

As an aside, I did go on to complete my first marathon in 2007 during residency. I continued to run because I was of the mindset to hold onto who I was in residency. People told me that the residency years would take "everything" away from me, but I wanted to keep my identity as an athlete. As for triathlon, I went on to complete my first full-distance Ironman triathlon in 2009. I am an Ironman. Just ask the voice of Ironman, Mike Reilly! When you identify as something, you become that thing.

Remember, when I talk to you about exercise, I'm talking about movement. You don't have to do a triathlon or a marathon. Your activity could range from some sit-ups in your living room to a 100-mile trail race. Your movement is *your* movement, but no matter what, it's time to move. Tap into that source energy because you cannot live Happy First without getting up and getting going.

# Chapter 9
# Relationships

The Happy First chapter on relationships is shorter than a lot of them. I won't profess to be an authority on relationship success, but I am an authority on relationships as a work in progress. A mentor of mine is a noticeably big proponent of "love always wins," and I can't disagree. When in doubt, love is the answer. Whether it's a friendship, a marriage, your child, or a coworker, kindness gets you further than nagging or anger. Much like allowing rather than fighting is the best way to achieve success. Every one of these people in your life has fears and hopes and dreams that you're lucky enough to be privy to as their confidante.

It behooves us to remember in any relationship that the other person is born of the same energy that we are. Even though they have a wildly different opinion or may be acting outright mean or cruel, this behavior has more to do with them being cut off from their connection to the Happy First energy rather than having anything to do with you.

One of the hardest lessons to learn is that it's better to be kind than right. Oh boy, do I like to be right. My boss and I spoke about six months ago about some work circumstances and I ended up saying to myself, "Maybe I don't know best." That statement carries on as a mantra for me. Do you know who *does* know best? That inner wisdom. That inner energy that I'm calling Happy First. The way of living that grounds you into a place of stability and infinite ability to give, is the place your words and actions should always flow from. This is how you create a life of peace and contentment. You open the channel for the energy to flow *through* rather than always having to tap into some reserve that is made by you. Giving from a shallow well is a recipe for failure in any relationship.

Any time you decide to come from a place where you're dipping into your reserve, you'll eventually start to ask what's in it for you. Once you start asking that question, it gets difficult to extricate yourself from that loop. But it can be done, and that's part of the focus of this book. I want to show you that there's an instantaneous way out.

Aside from instances of physical abuse—in which case you don't just need coaching and Happy First, you need a safe place to go—you will be amazed at the changes that can happen in a relationship when you give from an unlimited wellspring of love and faith and hope.

That is the crux of Happy First in relationships. The way I picture it is when you feel broken and it feels like your heart and soul are cracked open, that is a doorway through which your inner wisdom flows. It is in these times of desperation that you're likely to search for solace. If you tap into the Happy First energy, it can be immediate relief. You may need something like a grounding exercise in color. For example, you look outside and say, "The grass is green," "The clouds are gray," and so on. Then you progress to more complex statements such as, "I'm sitting on a hard bench." These things bring you back to yourself.

Connecting yourself to the world around you reminds you that you're not alone. You have a never-ending energy flowing through you. You may be asking yourself, "Well, how do I know I have energy flowing through me?" My simple answer to that is: because you're breathing. You are a manifestation of thought in this world. You are lucky enough to be able to interact with other people who are also manifestations of energy. We learn from them; we care for them, we love them. The most important thing we can do is love them. That might be my best piece of advice. Give more love today than yesterday. It doesn't get used up. You've got plenty.

# Chapter 10
# Puppies, Cats, and Caps Lock

In this chapter, let's talk about the things that happen that threaten your ability to live Happy First. Let's start with the little things. You set yourself up to come from a position of happiness and peace, and then suddenly, something annoys you. One of the most common things that happens to me is that my wonderfully supportive cuddly large cat hits the caps lock and types on my computer while I'm in a meeting. Sometimes, he'll also send these forceful messages in all caps to people in a professional meeting. The last time this happened, I started to laugh and termed this phenomenon "Bennie and the caps lock." Humor is always better. As another example, sometimes I'm journaling, deep into my mental process, and Bennie walks across my keyboard in front of my face, changes what I'm doing and interrupts my train of thought. All that serenity and insight I gained while writing my journal for the day seems to be gone. I realize this concern is insignificant. But in the moment, it bugs the crap out of me. Bennie and the caps lock can immediately disrupt the flow of energy that manifests itself as happiness. Not to be left out, Zipp, our other cat (who knocks on my sleep room door about 20 minutes after I go into the room, or meows incessantly for cat food, when there is food *in his dish*), doesn't play by my rules either.

Let me give you a canine concrete example. Over the past three years, we've adopted two puppies. The first, Terrwyn (nicknamed Wyn), is a Welsh terrier who looks like Angus the Airedale, our first dog who passed away a few years ago. Thankfully, Wyn is about a quarter of Angus's size. He's also known as the landscaper. He's eaten more rose bushes than I can count, snips the top off our sago palms; yes, I know they're poisonous—Wyn does not. The terrier is more robust than a little plant. He has also eaten two sets of patio furniture. At two years old, he finally seems to be, other than the sago palm fronds, calming down. Then, we got Jazmin the Hungarian vizsla. She's almost a year old. Vizslas are calm dogs, they said. Even with a terrier to wear her out, she's crazy. And she's vocal. She barks and sniffs and whines. My life is grand from a 10,000-foot view, and I have what some people call gold-plated problems. But I will tell you that whining dog is enough to make me chuck the entire Happy First concept. One more chewed piece of resin wicker in my backyard is enough for me to give up on the entire pursuit of self-improvement.

Although I'm using our beloved pets as examples of my day-to-day woes, I would offer them up as examples of opportunities. When a child comes to us, upset and angry, their need for attention at an inopportune time pushes our buttons. They are human and they should "know better." Animals don't have that capability. But, funny enough, neither do most humans. We're all selfish by nature. We all want what we want when we want it.

In all reality, these animals are our best examples of unconditional love. They let Happy First flow through because they don't have a choice. They don't share our preconceived notions and expectations of how life should go. They just are. That terrier will just go on chasing squirrels. The vizsla will go and chase the terrier. Bennie will follow me around, and Zippy, well he's just going to be Zippy. They don't have much of an agenda except to be happy and comfortable and have some fun. They don't walk across my keyboard to make me angry or to disrupt me delving into my self-improvement space to deprogram all the programming. They just want to be close. They want to give love. That's the beauty of pets. Well, it's also their curse. They don't understand that sometimes we *do* have an agenda.

So, why not let those pets that you have, or maybe even the people in your life, be a barometer for you? Why don't you let them alert you to the fact that maybe you aren't giving as much love and attention to yourself, or your spouse, or your children, or your coworkers, or your pets as you could be. Maybe you aren't allowing that Happy First energy to flow through. Maybe you aren't reminding yourself to stop and reconnect with that inner knowledge of what's right and true. Maybe that's why those pets are here. Maybe you have these certain pets so they can push you in a way that opens that old rusty door and lets the light in. Maybe that coworker got a job in your office not just to annoy you and be the bane of your existence, but to push you into a *new* existence. From a quantum physics perspective, that's how you flip to the new reality. In common language, something pisses you off enough that you change. Maybe you realize that you've always hated this job and you need to get out. Maybe that coworker has traits that you, in fact, have but cannot stand. Maybe those habits are the ones that drive you to alcohol, or food, or working too much overtime. Maybe your soul is asking for these people in your life so you can see a noticeably clear reflection of what you need to change. Maybe without being able to see it, you wouldn't change it. It might be too comfortable staying precisely as you are. It's the way you've always been, so it's what you know.

Just because something is your norm doesn't mean it's healthy. We as human beings need connection. Fear and self-righteousness and hurry and indecision and busyness all serve to cut the ties that bind. Those connections are necessary for us to give and receive energy. That's the energy that I've been talking about. That energy that comes through us was there before us; it will be there after us. We are human conduits. Our purpose is to enrich the lives of others, and, in the process, we cannot help but be enriched.

As a personal example, I had come up against a tipping point about ten years ago. I could not stand being inside my own head. I felt like I had no home, no place. I couldn't help but think that maybe I was born broken. I have two parents who loved me very much then and still do. But for some reason, I could not feel that. It's as if the lens cover on my camera were stuck on. Since that time, I've grown to understand this phenomenon because I've seen others that can't feel the love that clearly surrounds them. No amount of chiseling away at that lens cover makes them see. But what I discovered about a decade ago was that by creating my *own* home the people around me could not help but experience that sense of home as well.

One of my coworkers said that I was extremely hard to get along with for the first bit while I worked at my current job. Then something changed. She attributed it to my having my son. But it was more of me creating a home, which was something I did prior to our son being born. I believe that also played a part in his conception. He was in fact, invited. There was a place for him to go. There was emotional space and physical space for his soul to settle with ours. The coworker felt that "home" energy flow through me and perceived it as me being easier to get along with.

That time in my life was quite bizarre. It was as if I had been reborn. I saw things differently; I did things differently, I experienced things differently. I became a different person. Regrettably, I lost some of that insight when a few years later I picked up my fear again. I clutched it like an old threadbare blanket that provides no warmth but is oh-so-familiar. I am learning to forgive myself with dignity as I move beyond this fear once again. This road is uniquely mine, and your road will be uniquely yours.

I only hope to illustrate here that the things that annoy or shake you likely serve a purpose. No matter how bad you think things are right now, there's nothing that cannot be changed by allowing love to flow through.

These principles apply not just to everyday things but even to circumstances that seem insurmountable—like when a loved one is depressed and you cannot see how to help them (or when you realize you cannot fix them, as we are often wont to do), show them love, then show them more. You'll be amazed at the miracles that can happen when you create a safe space for them to grow that feels like home—maybe a home as they've never felt. Hope and faith and love are not just cute Sunday school lessons. They are real, experiential vibrations that change lives.

# Chapter 11
# Play

I know you're wondering, "What's the difference between exercise and play?" Well, those of you who know me know that I need a dedicated spot for my Marvel movies. So, here's where they go. Sure, exercise can be play. When we tell our kids to "play outside," we're traditionally talking about activity. However, I also consider screen time—video games, YouTube, and movies—play.

We connect through play as well as through giving and loving and providing. When I was young, my dad and I would connect when he would teach me things on the computer. I loved that time when he shared his love of programming and computers with me. I've learned from our son that play can be fun. Having fun and being peaceful aren't things I'm naturally good at. They're traits I've had to cultivate. When our son was little, he would ask me questions about the Sinister Six or who Iron Man was fighting in the books we would read, and I wouldn't know. Or he would ask me who a certain character was when we finished a Marvel movie. I didn't know, so I would look it up. Somehow through all the research I did to answer a child's wondering questions, I became completely enthralled with the Marvel cinematic universe. We read bedtime stories and we watch YouTube videos about character development and new movies coming out.

We learn about how Tony Stark went from a selfish creator of weapons to a devoted husband and father. With the passing of Chadwick Boseman, whom we know as Black Panther and King T'Challa, the door opened to speak of cancer and how, although he only had 43 years on this planet, his legacy of honor and putting forth his talents to create made him a true gift to this world. Even the actors that portray these superheroes become fixtures in our conversations. When Matthew makes a mistake such as interrupting, I can reinforce lessons that he's been taught in school by telling him, "We've got some red in our ledger" to quote Black Widow and explain how we need to wipe it out. He relates. He understands that people make mistakes and that they atone for those mistakes. By playing and watching seemingly frivolous entertainment, we learned that when you interrupt, you must apologize—not because someone told you to, but because it feels better in your soul. The more of those actions we take, but don't apologize for, the more we impede the flow of that inner wisdom and abundant energy.

And sometimes, the movies are just fun, which is an inherent benefit. By smiling, you open up that energy channel. By sharing time with your family to watch the Star Wars movies, you not only enhance your ability to live Happy First, but you also show your children and your loved ones how to do that as well. With every one of us who gets happier, the world becomes a better place.

We cannot scream at people to be happy. We cannot effectively create change by expecting people to act as we have chosen to. Nagging doesn't produce positive change. Begging and pleading blocks that Happy First energy very quickly, in the person you're nagging as much as in yourself. At our core, we all want to feel good. This is why you're reading this book. We want our lives to be better. We want our days to be better. We want to make more money. We want to be fitter. We want to have more peace. We want to wake up energized and go to bed satisfied. We want to be excited to live.

One of the simplest ways to cultivate this is to play. Take some time out of your day and read a contemporary romance. Pick up a Patricia Cornwell book and lose yourself. Rewatch the Marvel movies, all of them. No, I don't mean in one day. I do live in reality!

I spoke earlier of goals, and I talked about earning a degree or running a marathon or learning to sew or paint. But what if your goal is simply to stop being so serious? My husband jokes that I was born 35 years old. I can't disagree. I play more now than I ever have in my life. Oddly I've also accomplished quite a bit. Do I procrastinate? Yes, too much even for my own liking. But you know what? I get things done. I usually get stuff done on time. What that knowledge has taught me is that it's alright to loosen up a bit. And *gasp,* I can actually chill without using alcohol or food. I'm allowed to relax.

There are unfinished tasks right now, whether home, work or publishing tasks. And yet I still plan to watch a movie later. I'll go outside and take some of my fun apps and look at the stars. If I'm lucky it'll be one of the days of the International Space Station flyover. Those are excellent days. Sometimes I wave. They can't see me, but remember, we're connected. They can feel it. They know we're here and we see them. Just like your spouse knows you're there. Just like your child who's in school knows you're there. Recall what I discussed in the last chapter—

they feel that sense of home. Home is not created with money and toil alone. Home is creative play and love and forgiveness and welcome.

To help foster that connection, invite others to play. Sometimes their play might not be your play. Sometimes you may need to meet people where they are. People respond better to you going to them. I have a friend I love to run with. She runs at my pace, whatever it might be for that day, because she's grateful for my company and she's grateful to be moving. I'm not sure she understands the depth of my appreciation for her willingness to "play" with me. We don't set any land speed records, we don't solve the world's problems with our meandering conversations, but she plays with me, and for that I am truly grateful.

Something that happened during the quarantine of 2020 was a perfect example of a simple way to play. It was called #KindnessRocks. Adults and children alike painted rocks and placed them on sidewalks, paths, and front lawns as a message of love and kindness. Some of these creations have been extremely elaborate. There was one by the pond in our neighborhood that was the likeness of SpongeBob SquarePants. I've seen ladybugs, M&Ms, and elaborate scenes. My family painted palm trees and beach scenes. I saw thank-yous to veterans for Memorial Day. At the corner of our street is a purple swirly one that says, "good vibes." I take that one to heart.

The next street over has a rounded triangular rock that looked to someone like an alien head, so it's green now with alien eyes. It's fantastic! A few houses down there's another rock that looked like a shark opening its mouth, so now it is. All these rocks are play. They're also a way to spread kindness. Think about it: is anyone stopping you from painting a rock? Where do you get the kindness to put in the rock? What do you think it comes from? Do you create it? Nope. But it is abundantly available to you whenever you want it. All you must do is tap in.

Social media groups are another interesting form of play. Like-minded people are getting together to share their enthusiasm over a subject. It's not only productive, it's play. Play is much broader than the traditional constraints we attempt to place on it. It's not just board games or card games. It can be video games, or silly talks over dinner. Play can be appreciating the beauty of a flower. Whatever you enjoy, that puts a smile on your face and lets you tap into that inner wisdom, that's play.

## Smile and Play

# Chapter 12
# The Job Dilemma

Our son often asks me, "Mom, why do you have to go to work?" My response is usually something like "because I like to go to Disney World." That isn't the whole story, but I do love the land of Walt. Looking from a Happy First perspective, and knowing that my energy comes from a timeless energy present long before me, I know that I was drawn to my profession for a reason. I'm a full-time emergency medicine nocturnist. It suits me. From the outside, people look and think my job is difficult because I work nights, take care of sick patients, currently during a pandemic, take care of trauma patients, take care of trauma surgeons, and deal with end-of-life issues on a regular basis. The moms of children I know see it as difficult because I'm away from my family. I have an odd sleep schedule and a non-traditional eating schedule. I work nights and a lot of weekends. Again, it suits me. There are certainly times that I would like to work fewer shifts in a month, but I cannot imagine a time that I do not practice as an emergency medicine physician. Like we often feel toward relatives, I don't always *like* my job, but I always *love* it. I've worked extremely hard to earn my medical degree and train in emergency medicine. I continue to work hard to learn about my profession and help myself and my colleagues improve.

I do other things on the side, such as writing, or coaching, but no longer do I work in multiple emergency departments and have not for many years. I find that my mind gets scattered easily. This matters because complexity muddies the waters. The more complex my workout regimen is, for example, the more difficult it is for me to comply. The more moving parts you have to my nutrition plan, the more difficult it is for me to implement. To have that space in your life for that Happy First grounding energy to flow and be directed to your thoughts and actions, you need to structure your life to create space. I'm not talking about taking hours on end to sit and contemplate your navel. I mean that if it feels difficult for you to arrange multiple job schedules, you find a way to consolidate. Suppose your current occupation creates mental strain regarding the logistics of it. In that case, you can either clear that up internally, which is always what I would suggest first, or possibly seek a new occupation and or new place of employment. Beware, however, of the situation trap or geographic cure. Once you fix one negative external circumstance, it's like the mythical Hydra: two more pop up in its place.

Why *do* we need to work? The obvious answer is we live in the real world and the real world uses money as currency. But look at it more deeply. Some people live on a tenth of what you make, and others who live on ten times what you make. You know as well as I do that some of those people are happy and some are miserable, regardless of the income.

We do need to pay for things such as food and utilities and housing. But those specifics can vary widely. Taking time to dig into what matters to you, regarding your house for example, is the key to streamlining the *why* you need to work question. If you would prefer greater square footage and create more value through employment, that will settle well internally when implemented. But if your stress level climbs and you get cut off from that inner wisdom and happiness because of what you feel is a huge mortgage, you need to reevaluate your priorities. Taking time to find out what suits you is key.

Some people would rather live in a smaller house and work less or dine out less or have a different gym membership or reallocate savings than have what they perceive as stress from many moving parts. Another person can be just as happy in a house three times the size, working twice as much with 25 different memberships to manage. What others see as chaos gives them energy. Admittedly, those are also the people who are able to compartmentalize and structure their lives so they have support and much is automated. But no one circumstance can be prescribed for everyone. Sometimes, those who do not have jobs outside the home provide the most value in a family, even though they don't bring a monetary paycheck. When I speak of a job, there are times where it's not a direct earning of money, but more of a providing of a service. A parent who raises children creates space for their spouse to dedicate to work, for example.

Therefore, when you're asking yourself, "Why *do* I have to work?" the answer is not as simple as money. The answer is that we feel more fulfilled when we provide value to the world. When we allow that Happy First energy to flow through us via our hopes and dreams and actions, we put that energy into the world. To quote an aphorism used by John F. Kennedy, "a rising tide lifts all boats."

By providing services as a doctor, I put a certain energy

into the world. Ideally, it's a positive, productive, healing energy, although actual mileage may vary. Any service profession puts energy into the world. Anyone raising children, whether they work outside the home or not, put *huge* amounts of energy into the world. Each of us either channels that source energy or we get cut off and attempt to use our reserve. By the time you reach this point in the book, your energy is coming consistently from that place of Happy First. You've learned how to live Happy First and that gets translated into your work and home. You can provide more value, which coincidentally brings in more money, as the laws of the universe would have it. Allow yourself to simplify, follow what you truly wish to have and be, and continue to achieve success from an authentic place of abundance.

# Chapter 13
# Time in the Day

This topic made me want to rewrite the last chapter on work and jobs. I wanted to write it between shifts rather than on a day away from the hospital to elucidate that time is not always what we perceive. Many scientists share Albert Einstein's view that time is, in fact, a "stubbornly persistent illusion." I don't usually write between shifts because most days it feels like time is scarce. Although, on days like today I feel like I have all the time in the world.

Interestingly enough, in our human lifetime, time *is* technically scarce. Our years on Earth are relatively short, although we often act as if they're long. If we see time as abundant, we tend to waste it. That also seems to be the antithesis of living Happy First. There is some art and discovery to making that balance work.

If you live by the concepts we've been discussing, you've been living from an ideology that we always have enough. Living Happy First means carrying out your days from the viewpoint that you are always enough. Addressing being enough appears to make this chapter somewhat of a paradox. In order to live with a time abundance mindset, you've got to firmly entrench yourself in the present moment. That's extremely difficult when you're planning goals or taking steps to reach those goals.

This came to light today when I talked to my husband

about learning a different language. He told me that he'd like to, but since he is now enrolled in higher education again, that must take all priority over other intellectual pursuits. Instead of seeing this as a scarcity, this relative lack of time shows importance. He has all the time in the world to accomplish what he is guided to pursue. When goals and dreams are examined in the light of prioritizing, this concept makes more sense.

As the philosopher Peter McWilliams cleverly noted, "You can have anything in life you really want—but you can't have everything in life you really want. Decide." Our goals and dreams and thoughts often become overwhelming when they're piled on top of one another. We can succeed at our passions, and it helps to have a method of sorts. A wise person once told me to make a list of 20 things I wanted to do in the next year, and then cross off numbers 3 through 20. When you put all those tasks into one moment, they get too big.

Say your two relatively immediate goals are to put on muscle and complete your current coursework for this 8-week block. (I'm borrowing that from my husband). That means your dinner is getting larger, and you'll have to sit down and do some homework. Are you currently doing work or are you making dinner? Even if you only have two tasks at hand, in the moment you must choose one. You have plenty of time to add a second serving of dinner. That particular task takes a minimal extra time investment. Does that mean your classwork isn't as important? No. You must set your priority right *now*. The only thing you can do in this moment is exist, and that is enough. It is more than enough. Do one thing right now. Do that thing, then do the next thing. All your goals have become reality before you know it, and somehow, you had plenty of time.

## Choose Your Own Adventure

This critical component to success is winning the moment. The only way we can truly get things done is in the right now. You can only eat well right now. You can only choose to nurture your body right now. You can't eat well tomorrow because tomorrow doesn't exist. The only way to make an impact on tomorrow is to live from a perspective of "I have everything I need right now to create the positive change." From a nutrition or fitness perspective, the only way to create tomorrow's athletic ability is to take action today.

As a person who naturally spent her life in overwhelm, it has been an interesting shift to move into a space of understanding that thought creates my overwhelm and *not* my circumstances. Everyone has plenty of things they want to do. And I know most of you are saying "but I *have* to do the laundry." A few perspectivists out there change their wording to incorporate "I get to" or "I choose to." You don't have to empty the garbage, clean your house, take the kids to school, or go to work. Those are all choices. Each choice has consequences to both doing and not doing it. You can sit on the couch and do nothing for as long as you choose. Eventually someone will come in and take you away on a waterproof tarp if you sit long enough. You prefer not to have a dentist drilling into your tooth enamel, so you brush your teeth. You prefer not to have the burden of 30, 40, 100 pounds of extra fat on your body, so you eat some vegetables. You prefer to take a clean breath of fresh air, so you quit smoking. Everything in life is a choice.

The key is to make those choices from a place of joy and abundance and happiness—from the energy that flows through everything, including you—rather than making a choice based on fear or lack or feeling rushed. Choice in the moment made in the service of joy or happiness always wins. The actions based on fear or lack always feel like burdens rather than like freedom. Indeed, the fear is there, but you aren't deciding on action based on running from that feeling. You decide to feed into your higher good.

Ironically, true freedom is born of discipline. You must create routines and compartmentalization to create the space for spontaneity. To have the freedom of mind, you must have both a momentary perspective and an overall perspective for your life; you must see your big picture. You've got to consider the moment at hand and how that moment changes who you are. I honestly believe our purpose in life is to align ourselves with the person we were meant to be. Step into that role. Many of the messages we carry from childhood via intent or perception take us far away from our true nature. Now, we can learn to be adults and live life on life's terms. We are meant to open the door to that energy of abundance and see not only our true nature but also how to take our life into that space.

In the work chapter, I talked about external "solutions" such as getting a new job versus getting a new perspective. In the nutrition chapter, I talked about discovering what works for you both in the moment and long-term. I spoke about relationships and how giving love is always the answer. In this chapter, I'm addressing your relationship with yourself and with time.

## Chapter 13 - Time in the Day

We see time as linear, but it is anything but. Our thoughts create so much about our existence that we can't comprehend. The quantum physicists out there can get a better grasp, along with the enlightened ones. But for most of us, we're just looking to marry the day-to-day grind with the attainment of the potential we can feel is inside.

Often, you'll hear that happiness is your birthright. That always sounds pompous and egotistical to me. I prefer to describe reality in terms of happiness being our true nature. You aren't entitled to happiness. You *are* happiness. Happiness isn't something we must fight or argue for; it's merely present. There's no denying that your baseline is one of love and light and happiness. The challenge is to accept that. And by accepting that your true nature is happiness, you must then accept that all the overwhelm and all the negativity that inserts itself into your days, comes from *you*. It comes from the way you've learned to do things. The feeling of overwhelm or negativity(or at its extreme, hatred) is not you. These emotions are how you learned to handle what appeared to be external circumstances. Your feelings are all thought-created.

So, what next? I'll get into this more in part three, but let me give you a bit of introduction now. You have a day where life just feels like too much to handle, too many things to do, too many places to be, too many whatevers. That picture is fake. You might find yourself in the thought loop that has you convinced that you don't have enough love to give or time for yourself. But you've got plenty of it. We addressed this point. The solution is not to do anything extra. There is nothing to add to your task list. You may need to take some things away, but in reality, a shift in perspective is universally more effective.

Time seems to expand when you enjoy your task. That aspect of creation is totally within your control. Imagine taking whatever task it is, and smiling while thinking of it, or starting it. When you're faced with an unwanted chore, take a deep breath and allow yourself to begin from a place of being settled. Take a moment and be grateful for one thing that enables you to perform the task. Be thankful your arms allow you to carry the laundry basket, or that you have a washer in your home. Feel the fabric as you fold the clothes. Overwhelm comes from fear. When you come from gratitude instead, fear dissolves. Fear of lack of time, fear of lack of love, fear of lack of money, all of it compounds.

Living in abundance is the only way to start. Any time a task is born of obligation or threat, those emotions multiply as well. It may take a dedicated effort, in the beginning, to mentally check up and say, "This bores me" instead of "I hate this." Soon you can see the truth in "I choose to be bored by this." Then think about the task with gratitude and stability. "I am so grateful that I can do my laundry in my home," or something similar that resonates in you. The mindset is a simple shift, but one that changes everything. Once you start to do this on a reflexive basis, you've changed. Sometimes, it feels like the world has changed, without changing your external environment at all. Wait, and watch.

# Chapter 14

# Kindness

One of the big movements today is self-care and self-kindness. I have a revelation for you. Sometimes being kind to yourself doesn't mean what you think it means. Sometimes, it means working hard or feeling some discomfort. Kindness doesn't always mean carving out time for yourself isolated from your family; it could mean giving your time to others when you feel like you don't have any to give. That, too, is being kind to yourself. Many pop-culture references will lead us to believe that the only way to employ self-kindness is meditation, massage, time alone reading, indulging in food or alcohol, or avoiding work. Often, *doing* the work is the kindest thing you can do for yourself.

Counterintuitive as it may be the kindest thing you can do for yourself might even look like stern discipline. Tough love, in a way. For example, about 300 days before writing this, I embarked on a "run every day journey." I get out and run every day. There are days when I don't feel well, or don't have the mental fortitude or maybe have a niggling beginning of an injury. That day's run might consist of a two-minute jog with walking after. But I run—every day. I am a person who runs every day. Over those 300 or so days, I have reinvented myself. I don't just work out every day, I *run* every day. Does this make me a runner? Nope, I was a runner before. I've been doing running races since

2008 or so. Does my speed make me a runner? Nope. What makes me a runner is what I define as a runner.

What matters most to me is that I see myself as an active person. I run every day. I'm an athlete. That is kind. That helps me develop clarity in the things that I do every day. There are many days that I don't want to run or walk. I want to sit with another cup of coffee, yet I go outside and I move. That is kindness. Some will say that is rigid and inflexible. I define what running is. And as I said, because I define it, and some days it includes a significant amount of walking, I continue to be who I am. I continue to grow into the person I'm meant to be. That is what I mean by living Happy First.

A lot of my analogies and lessons come from activity and food. I've discussed my disordered eating patterns in the past, and one thing I always struggled to define for myself was food abstinence. My sponsor has been ever-so-patient with me for more than 15 years, and I've asked her over and over again what she would define as food abstinence. She has told me to work with a nutritionist, which I have—more than once. A lot of my nutrition ideas came from this process. My attempts at freedom from overeating have included many different externally imposed definitions of food abstinence or healthy eating. Honestly, none worked. The only periods of freedom from food obsession I've had were not on a "diet plan."

Recently I was introduced to a concept of *internal* definitions of bingeing that coincides strongly with my individual designation of success. Glenn Livingston, psychologist, and founder of www.neverbingeagain. com, suggests in his book of the same title that you must define *your own* plan of eating. When you sit and you calmly examine those food behaviors that may not make you overweight but create mental strife and hardship, you must avoid those behaviors and foods at all costs. Like someone with an allergy, you must learn to define yourself in terms of those things that cut you off from that Happy First energy. You cannot eat those things or in those ways. You must employ habits and processes that maintain your connection to your inner wisdom and inner knowing. Oddly, these paths of kindness look like rules to others. But remember, the best way to freedom is through discipline. The best way to live Happy First is by creating a structure in a framework that might look to someone else like rigid rules but feels to you like flying.

Kindness is both subjective and objective. For those of you who reference the Bible or other religious text, there are definitions of kindness that resonate. As we tell our son, it's okay to be angry; it's not okay to be mean. Of course, external measures of kindness are to be followed, but I believe those stem from internal practices. Read ten different websites, and you'll see that self-care ranges from pedicures to drunken nights out with friends. If we sit with ourselves for a moment, we can see that social interaction is essential. But I'm not sure I'll ever believe that oblivion is truly kind to yourself or others. Losing yourself in food or drink or shopping to excess or gambling or indiscriminate sexual encounters is never kind in the long run. I broach some immutable truths that are uncomfortable and must be faced head on to overcome.

Living Happy First doesn't mean always sitting in this marshmallow place of bliss. Sometimes it means being uncomfortable. Sometimes it means realizing that kindness has elements of pain. Sometimes self-kindness means that you push yourself and do hard work. This is the paradox of progress and becoming who you were always meant to be. There is discomfort that must be tolerated through your metamorphosis to carve away the old garbage. Michael Neill, in his audio program, *Effortless Success*, talks about how we are all diamonds who get covered in horse shit, then slap on some nail varnish to make ourselves look better. Instead, all we needed to do was wash off the shit.[3] In other words, that beauty is always there, immutable. This is Happy First. You don't have to imagine that you're a good person underneath. You don't have to imagine that you're a light, loving, active person. That is who you are. You must let that energy flow through and let that person be discovered—allowing over forcing.

When I use the word kindness, it doesn't mean letting yourself off the hook. Within the principles of Happy First, kindness means keeping yourself *on* the hook. You look closely to see what's important to you and take action accordingly. Seeing what's important will allow you to define yourself in a manner consistent with what you are both meant to be and also what you already are. Those rules and discipline are what allow the beautiful expression of that person.

---

3  Michael Neill, Effortless Success: How to Get What You Want and Have a Great Time Doing It, Read by the author, January 1, 2008, CD.

# Chapter 15
# Conversations

Learning to talk to yourself and others is crucial to your internal and external success. I'm not a big fan of hard personal conversations, although I have them with patients and families almost daily at work. Death and dying are difficult topics, and it's an honor to have these conversations even through illness. Yet, when I'm at home or with the people I love, it can be challenging for me to speak my mind and be honest. I'm sure some of you feel the same way. Fear often drives a reluctance to have open conversations. You may be afraid of rejection or you might worry about what will happen if you change your mind shortly after you communicate. For me, it's taken a great amount of practice in letting go of those fears and allowing myself to run the risk of being "wrong" for me to get comfortable having hard conversations with friends and family.

As difficult as it is to have conversations with others, we have some of the hardest conversations with ourselves. Sometimes facing your biggest fears or admitting to yourself that maybe you don't know best can be hard to stomach. But these conversations are necessary to crack open your shell, so to speak, to let that Happy First energy flow through and allow true growth.

Oftentimes, the conversations we have with ourselves

and others change over time. That's because people grow and change, always. For a long time, I thought we weren't allowed to change. I felt I had to set a goal, commit to it, and away we went. But I've accepted that change is a necessary part of life. Nothing in life is stagnant. If you need to, change the direction you were heading, even in the middle of a tough conversation. If the shift occurs with kindness, it shows you or the person involved that you're willing to be real, rather than compromise your integrity.

At times you may ask yourself what your goal of the conversation is. Maybe you need to make a career decision with the input of friends or family. It's possible that you need to win someone over to your opinion. Or you might need to foster love and cohesiveness. To reiterate key concepts from earlier, no matter your goal, always come from a place of love and remember that words matter. If you want to have real, honest conversations, you must settle in without fear of loss or rejection. You must listen to—and accept—what people say, most notably our loved ones. From that point, everyone involved is able to take the space of their own Happy First energy. Although this energy comes from the same source, we each have our own path and our own internal knowing. That's why there's not only one right way, not even only one right way for you. But there is one source for *all* our right ways. When we listen and speak from this space of Happy First, the tough conversations become kinder, softer, and more productive.

# Speak Kindly

As we get older, ideally, we make better decisions. Or we make all new wrong ones. Either way, the beauty of our human existence is sharing. We enrich our lives by learning to have the conversations with ourselves to open those channels. That way that we can then show up with other people. Imagine showing up *for real* with your children and your spouse by having an open and honest conversation without—or despite—fear. Imagine showing your true self to your aging parents.

When you have meaningful conversations, the feelings get big. Earlier, I likened that to the image of walking around bleeding from your eyeballs. But it's more accurate to say it's like walking around without skin. Everything is raw. Everything feels ten times as potent as it did the day before. The difference is that, once you learn to show up as yourself, you don't wish for that raw pain to dissipate immediately. You don't long for blissful numbness. You appreciate that the intensity of feeling shows you that you're truly alive.

When we have real conversations with people who matter to us, and let them into our world, we create change. We show people that they matter enough to present ourselves to them in all our unique individuality. Now that you know where you come from and where your real strength lies, there's no going back. You have a deep, deep knowing that the energy that flows through you, the energy that created you, is your life force and is expressed uniquely through you. If we don't share this uniqueness in speech and cadence and meaning, we don't share our true selves.

Our expression through words and heartfelt thoughts not only changes our world, but it also changes the world of those we love—for the better. Others now have the freedom to show up as their naked selves without fear.

When I talk about this with people, many of them tell me that whenever they share something somebody gets mad at them. Well, if everyone gets defensive when you speak what you think is your truth, I need you to take a step back and consider that this may *not* be your truth. You may be speaking your fear or using words that cultivate fear in others. You may be choosing to deaden the raw feelings by building up walls instead of boundaries. Boundaries are loving, they flex, they have space. Boundaries stand and sway like a palm tree in the storm. Walls are built to keep out the pain, but they eventually crumble. Walls cut you off from the Happy First energy. Learn to sway like the palm tree. Learn to express yourself and reach out, because when you reach out from that place of pure love and kindness, you create real change within yourself and your environment. But you cannot force growth, in yourself or in another. True change must come from within. The best progress comes from your inner wisdom and energy. Every time you tap into the flow of source that is timeless, infinite, and immutable, you show your body and your mind the path to peace.

You will have arguments, see differences of opinion, and encounter negative circumstances. You also will learn to stand like the palm tree. You learn to weather the storm. You learn to bend with grace. You learn to hold your head high and stand as yourself. Like the palm tree, you know no different way to be.

I implore you, start having productive conversations. If

you want help to get to this point, head to LiveHappyFirst.com and sign up for coaching. Even one session may be groundbreaking. Start opening up in small statements to the ones you love. Just let them see you. Let that Happy First energy shine through. Be diligent in remembering it's there. Allow other people to see the light through you. One by one, we all can bask in the warmth of the Happy First energy.

# Happy First

# Part 3

# Chapter 16

# Change the Program

In part 2, I discussed a multitude of areas of your life where you can employ Happy First. I also included examples of how I've chosen to do things. Now, I'm going to wrap up by bringing specific illustrations back to more general guidelines.

The only way to really change how you do things and the way you exist within the world is to change your program. Our thoughts and our actions all stem from old tapes that we play and old scripts that we follow. I'd love to be able to say that changing the program is easy, but, instead, I can tell you it is absolutely possible. As Michael Neill has asserted in his 2008 audio program *Effortless Success,* "It takes effort to become effortless at anything."[4] On the start of your Happy First journey, it feels like every statement, every text reply, takes an inordinate amount of thinking. This process gets more efficient with time.

There are two schools of thought in changing your life experience: Inside Out and Outside In. I subscribe wholeheartedly to the Inside Out methodology. By changing your internal environment, the outside world changes. At the outset, your view is the first aspect to shift. We know that the immutable energy of Happy

---
4    Michael Neill, Effortless Success: How to Get What You Want and Have a Great Time Doing It, Read by the author, January 1, 2008, CD.

First is stable. We know that our thoughts, although they appear fixed, are, in fact, changeable. By this logic, we must change our thoughts to change our existence.

Ironically, sometimes the quickest way to change your thoughts is to change your actions, and oftentimes, the best way to change your internal program is to do something different. Notice, I didn't say "think about something differently." A lot of this book references thought processes, but we are after tangible results—changes in observable circumstance. Let's go back to the familiar runner example. Say you'd like to change your program that you're not a runner. You have always just "known" that you're not a runner. To some people, that means you're not a fast runner. To other people, that means you can't run more than a mile. To yet another group, not being a runner means you never run. The definition is not set in stone, so your job is to make it your own.

Part of changing the program is defining what success is. You must outline exactly what something would look like so that you, as well as a casual observer, would agree. In the runner example, I run daily—that makes me a runner. For me, distance doesn't matter. If you define yourself as a runner, you may have completed a 5K race, or run track in high school, or whatever you define as a "runner." It matters not what the definition is, but it must be something that resonates with you. It's a clear checkbox. If I looked at your week's activities and you told me your definition of a runner, I could also say, "Yes, you did those things."

Clarity always helps. With relationships, this isn't as simple as a checkbox. But if you desire to build a more cohesive family unit, coming home from work angry every day and yelling at your spouse wouldn't support that goal. If you need to decompress from work, and you want to show love to your family, you could set an objective such as "make connection the top priority in any conversation I have at home." It's a bit more nebulous but still serves to change each interaction at the outset.

When you start building on smaller victories, you learn to trust yourself. Realizing that you have this unlimited source of pure positive energy bubbling up through you and combining that with the knowledge that you're able to carry out the directives your brain receives from that wellspring is an enormously powerful combination. *That* is how you change the program. Tap into the energy; let it guide your actions. In making yourself a conduit, you've got to lay down the wiring before you can expect that energy to flow through.

With our human minds, the wiring process is usually done best through words and actions. This combination is potent. Taking external input and circumstances as motivation helps open that door. That argumentative family member is exactly what you need to provide the impetus and opportunity to change. That is the time to say something different, kinder. During the tantrum is the time to hug your child rather than yell.

## Always More Hugs

We all could use a little program upgrade. You picked up this book because you feel this need for a reboot. If you were already tapped into this never-ending source of creativity and love, you wouldn't be wondering why all these external circumstances look great, but you still don't feel happy. You may not feel fulfilled. You've got the spouse, the house, the dog, the kids, and the white picket fence—but where is the bliss?

Here's where I push you to look on the inside. That's where all good work is done. Connect with that deeper knowing regardless of your external circumstances before you decide to attempt life changes by asking your spouse to do things differently, or changing jobs, or doing any number of things that are at best a temporary fix. Before you distract yourself with a new hobby or new challenge, get yourself on a good footing—with those conversations with yourself. We've been raised in an Outside In society. We put metaphorical Band-Aids® on cancerous thoughts. Without the knowing that comes from this internal energy, the external trappings become meaningless. With the grounding in Happy First, any outside circumstances take on new meaning.

I can tell you that the devil on your shoulder (or maybe it's the angel) is going to come back at me and say, "but you don't know my boss, he's a … " And I bet that voice could list a variety of other circumstances that tell me I'm wrong.

Here is where I ask you to take a leap of faith. For you to fully enjoy some aspects of your boss, for example, you must come from a place of love and light and giving. There are no two ways about it. From Mahatma Gandhi to Viktor Frankl, there are authors much more eloquent than I who espouse this idea. Your world is what you make of it. William Shakespeare eloquently quipped, "There is nothing either good or bad, but thinking makes it so."

By changing the thought process and changing the

program, you keep that Happy First channel open. Just let that light flow through. And once that light comes on in the room, in your mind, you see things differently.

Some state changers, such as meditation, have been proven effective. Most of these involve movement, and I'll go through a long list in chapter 23. Stand up straight. Smile. Find colors in your environment. Feel your feet on the ground. Take a deep breath. Take a drink of water. Feel the sun on your face. Taste a piece of fruit. Move to a chair outside. Notice, though, that as a human being, most of the state changers use your senses, whether it's your traditional five senses or in the sense of proprioception when you move. Neural feedback literally changes the way your brain is working. If you're depressed, don't stay inside a dark house all day. If you're tired, rest; do not drink or eat as a substitute. Change the program.

Notice when the words that you tell yourself are simply untrue. Watch out for those "always" and "never" bombs. When your brain says, "I will always feel this way," it lies. When your brain says, "I will never be happy again," it lies.

What are some things you can do today to change your program? A good first step is to look at labels you use for yourself: fat, thin, young, old, fast, slow, a procrastinator, a go-getter. Those are all relative terms, not absolute. There's not much place in a Happy First life for those words by themselves. Instead, we need to start rethinking our words. Use terms such as leaner. I'm leaner than I used to be. I work hard for that. I take a bit more time to rest before I get things done. It doesn't hurt anyone when you're kind to yourself. It certainly doesn't hurt you if you forgive yourself with dignity. Those around you will almost certainly respond favorably. Repeatedly reframing the words in your head is the second aspect to changing the program. The bodily action just makes it faster and easier. There are no situations that cannot be improved by coming from a place of love and joy and kindness.

# Chapter 17
# Admiration

In almost every circumstance there's someone who has succeeded at the endeavor you aspire to. Somebody out there did it first. In all reality, it's more like a hundred people, or even thousands. If one can, **you** can. We feel so alone and so unique in our troubles, yet we can easily find many people who have had our "problem" and found a solution. The good thing is that we're all individual. You can take parts of each of the solutions you find to suit yourself. Find examples of people who've created a positive life for themselves after tragedy or suboptimal circumstances. Read accounts of people who changed their lives from pessimism to optimism. Fill your brain with good words from audiobooks, podcasts, and interviews. Read success stories that resonate with you. Find business teachers who've created the business you want to create. Find forums of people who've successfully conquered the obstacles you know you'll have to conquer on the way to your dream.

Many years, ago my husband and I both decided to change careers from athletic trainers to physicians. At that time, I didn't know anything about getting in and going to medical school. So, I spent a lot of time on studentdoctor.net asking people questions. These forums were so helpful during premed prerequisites, the application process, and residency applications. When I had information to share,

I got back on to help others. I knew that, for hundreds of years, people have been becoming physicians. Since the advent of the internet, aspiring physicians have hopped on these forums to show others the way. I used their knowledge and experience to help light my path. As you succeed, you assist others and bring that light to the forefront. Like a candle that lights another candle, it doesn't extinguish, instead it begins to light the entire room. Most of the people who've achieved similar aspirations, even if it's a positive daily outlook or more energy in the morning, are more than willing to share their methods of attainment.

This inspiration and instruction doesn't need to be via direct contact. You can read books or blogs, or hire a coach or a teacher, or pay for organized instruction. You can ask clergy, neighbors, or friends of friends. Stand in awe and admiration for what others have created. Then, create your own version.

## Be You Today

This is a crucial aspect of following another's footsteps. You're rarely able to follow the entire path. There will be cracks in their sidewalks, or their path may not be wide enough for you and your family to travel. Such was the case with my husband and I going to medical school together. We needed to follow couples who applied. We were unique in our circumstances of being married and a bit older, so that presented additional "challenges" or more correctly, specificities.

When you emulate someone who has achieved a physical

## Chapter 17 - Admiration

feat such as an Ironman, you could follow the exact same training plan, but still not have equivalent results. You are you. Although we do have many common struggles, at the end of the day you create your version of your success. That's why I called this chapter "Admiration" rather than "Imitation." We don't want to be other people. We want to first tap into that Happy First energy, and then want to keep that conduit open so we can channel and live by the principles. After that, we want to go out and do our thing. You are headed toward a fantastic version of yourself. You as a calm, peaceful, loving human!

When you cut yourself off from that Happy First energy, you just don't feel like yourself. You feel like an imposter. When I say admiration, I'm not talking about envy. Jealousy has no place here. If someone goes on a vacation you'd love to take, you can either take that vacation or not. That's unrelated to anyone else's travel plans. If you discover that you don't have enough time or money to travel to the exotic destination your Facebook friend visited, you have choices. You either make the time, get the money, or don't go. Your success has nothing to do with other people's accomplishments.

When you admire someone, you look at her accomplishments and think, "Wow, I'd like to do that." The sentiment is more of an "I wonder if I can?" If you interject the negativity of jealousy or judgment, that cuts you right off from that Happy First energy. The light that inspires you to make a difference and make these things happen is hidden, and it appears that you're in the dark.

You're not. It's all appearances. But you need to be aware of these choices because when those emotions cut you off, it makes it harder to get anything done.

The thought tornado also interrupts the flow of this energy. Your brain escalates. You start borrowing problems (stop thinking about the sister who needs to get a better job or the latest newsworthy crime against someone you do not know). You make poor decisions if you're able to make any at all. It's like operating your life impaired. Why not just turn the light on? In the middle of negativity, flip open to chapter 23 and do some state changers. Anything you can do to get yourself closer to, or smack dab in the middle of, that happy hot spot will work. You'll find your easiest, fastest way to that Happy First energy, and you'll stay there—that's what I mean by living Happy First.

Go out there and find some role models. Find two…or ten! Find some people whose characteristics you like, or maybe even just the way they did one certain thing. The people you admire, you admire for a reason. They don't resonate with you by chance. They resonate with you because their energy resonates with yours. That's why admiration isn't jealousy or envy. Admiration includes synchronicity. Admiration is incorporating a bit of someone's energy or knowledge or experience or hope into your path.

If you need more concrete help in finding people to look up to, you may even want to consider a support group or online group where you have direct access to people who have similar trials and tribulations in your choice of journey. As I said in the relationship chapter, we are made to interact.

We aren't put on this earth to be alone. We're born to parents; we have friends and coworkers and families and neighbors and teachers and students with whom we travel the world. We crave the connection even when we're better at isolating. Even if being alone seems like your true nature, you'd be surprised once you open the channels for energy flow. Finding people to mentor you and guide you through complicated processes might be the first way you can initiate connection. Once you start to connect, the ability to weave your energies together grows. Mentorship is no small feat on either end. It takes a tremendous amount of openness and honesty to both give and receive emotion. That interaction may give more than you receive, and you may never feel the extent. Ask any parent or teacher. Our son gives me so much more than I feel I give, and that's why I work to stay in that Happy First space.

# Chapter 18
# Path of Least Resistance

When you look at nature, life flows downhill. Things follow the easiest path. A flower grows toward the sun. Water flows through the channel that it has produced. So how does that path get created? Investment. You must put energy in to push the ball up the hill. When you picture a tree growing toward the sun, it's drawn toward the potent source of energy the sun provides. We must first invest in putting down roots and then opening up to the energy flow. We must use that energy that comes underneath us, that Happy First energy, and be a conduit into the world.

We take the path of least resistance by being like the Colorado River in the Grand Canyon. We start with a small stream and over time and patience and diligence, we create a vast magnificent natural wonder. We make a larger and larger open space for that Happy First energy to flow. Initially, it feels like we're pushing the ball up the hill, but once we plug into that energy source, we are taking the path of least resistance. Inspired action is on a different wavelength than forced motivation.

Think about applying this to relationships. Which version of you do you think your spouse is going to be most attracted to? Is it the version that nags to do the same task over and over again? Or is it the one who realizes what's important, picks up the errant socks, and greets their spouse with a smile, overjoyed they came home safely? When you put forth positive energy, that energy has no choice but to create positivity as it flows through you. You become that path of least resistance for positivity.

Picture a frustrating situation at work. There's a protocol at the office that you disagree with, and you feel it makes your job harder. You could work to change the protocol, by perhaps going for an administrative position or lobbying with your coworkers to convince your boss of whatever it is that you need to change. That's a large amount of energy expended on your part to push the ball up the hill. What if you opened yourself up to the possibility that there's a chance to work within the protocol differently? What if you could carry out the required task within the current rule structure in such a way that it felt better to you? Maybe this means preparing differently for the task or arranging a meeting differently? There are infinite choices to change the situation without changing your company's entire infrastructure. This process still requires an energy investment, but in a different way. Work smarter, not harder. Go about any dilemma by affecting internal change first rather than modifying every external circumstance to make things go your way.

Look at your relationships with your pets or your children. Look at how they react. Getting angry and screaming at them to do things may make them get the task done, but at what cost? Screaming at people creates fear, intimidation, and false leadership. Keep in mind that people will follow the path of least resistance, which is avoiding punishment or bad feelings. Why not provide them with a path of least resistance that involves love and kindness? You can't help but create that environment of love and kindness within yourself by delivering it to them.

How about something as commonplace as fat loss or fitness? When you make yourself results-focused, consider it equivalent to a flower growing. Like a tree, a flower doesn't grow because you scream at it or throw food at it; it grows because it absorbs the energy from its environment and grows toward it. Popular culture would have us believe that the best way to change physique or health or fitness is via a rigid diet or food plan or exercise regime. In reality, creating an environment, as I discussed in both the activity and nutrition chapters, in which you *become* that person, genuinely establishes the path of least resistance. It's a subtle shift in perspective, but the most important one to live a life grounded in Happy First.

A lot of the resources published today emphasize that you need to be happy with who you are physically, regardless of physical condition. I don't think the two have to be exclusive. You can be fully aware that you have health concerns or potential health concerns based on your eating habits or body habits or lack of activity, *and* have the desire to change those, come from a place of Happy First. You tap into that energy and create a beautiful change out of love and self-kindness and positivity rather than employing "ten steps to a better booty," which will get you nowhere. Except for maybe an expensive treadmill you can hang your clothes on. It appears that the path of least resistance would be to just get it over with and lose the weight, for example. Anyone who's ever done this—and judging by statistics, that's most of us—knows that the changes you make by white-knuckling through it rebound with a vengeance. You don't want to create a fit person; you want to *be* a fit person.

This is why I work with clients on both an individual and

group basis. One on one, I can delve into each person's particular situation. In a group, a fair number of issues come up repeatedly, so when one person asks, another nods in agreement. We connect and learn from each other.

You want to be that palm tree growing tall toward the sun with a strong base, with the ability to bend in a storm and not break, and the functionality to have all your leaves cut off and grow an entirely new layer quickly and with purpose and beauty. You don't want to be a stick. You want to be dynamic and energetic. The path of least resistance for us in our human bodies is one of movement and flow. Once we open ourselves up to this ever-present energy and live from it, every day gets more enjoyable. Even if you're not at your "goal," that doesn't mean you don't enjoy every day in the process. Because in the process of becoming, you are already being.

When I talk about being yourself, what I have in mind is reminiscent of the aphorism, "Life isn't about finding yourself. Life is about creating yourself." When you create yourself, you are more like an artist that chisels away all that old programming, creating cracks in the marble that allow that infinite energy to flow through. Your creation is you allowing your true nature to shine through. Taking the path of least resistance initially might feel like going straight up a mountain. It's a change. It's like taking a left and not having road signs. The path was always there, you just weren't on it. By regularly touching base with that pure positive light and energy, you stay on that path and it quickly becomes the path of least resistance. Every day, you become closer to the person you're meant to be.

# Chapter 19

# Doubt Is Inevitable

Believing in ourselves doesn't come naturally to all of us. We second guess our decisions. We find guilt and shame in our outcomes. Guilt is useful — shame, not so much. Learn and move on. After what I would consider a significant negative patient event, my boss said, "You gotta let that shit go and move on. You're human."

You are here. There's nowhere to *get to*. There is no finish line and there is no linear path. You might have stumbling blocks every day, or every hour, or sometimes every minute. You might need to create a practice habit to learn to step into that Happy First place almost effortlessly. A daily practice is particularly valuable initially, when it seems like this is a massive shift. It's not much of a shift at all. It's just coming home.

Doubt in your path is inevitable. Living Happy First doesn't mean you wake up tomorrow and everything is hunky-dory. Living Happy First means you wake up tomorrow and you know there's a good, solid way to be. You know there's a place that you can always return to that offers all the solace you need. This place offers all the joy available to all of us in the world at all times. Life is sure to throw you some curveballs that make you doubt this, but just because you doubt it doesn't mean it isn't true.

When the doubt comes, move quickly through your shock. You knew it was coming, and you know it's coming again. The doubt is just another reminder that you're human. Welcome. Your mind is going to ask, "Is any of this real? Can I really live in a place of contentment?"

My challenge to you is to ask yourself: all that programming and garbage you lived in before, is that real? What is reality? Your thoughts create your world. So, when you doubt, expect it. You were waiting for it. But like that tall palm tree, when the hurricane came, it wasn't surprised. It knows that it lives in a world with hurricanes. It stood tall and strong and let the storm pass by. The storm always passes by. There will be new storms with new names and they'll pass by as well. Life and energy flow. You're part of that energy; you came from that energy, and you'll return to that energy. While you take this human form, you have a gift of being able to embrace that energy, channel it, and share it with others. You use it in your relationships, whether that relationship is with your coworkers or your children or your mind and body. What a fantastic opportunity we must use our world and our language to convey what we're becoming and what we are. We can show people by example the goodness that is present in all of us and in all circumstances.

Next time the doubt comes, welcome it. You are ready. You know what to do. Stand firm in your space. You're here to create your own version of greatness in the world.

# Chapter 20

# Fear Is Expected

Perhaps even more significant than doubt is fear. Many of us don't remember a time without worry. Maybe you had a perfect childhood, and the fact that people have chronic daily fears makes no sense to you. If so, be grateful. For those of us on the fear side of that seesaw, sometimes we sit in the thought tornado of irrational fear or in a state of complete paralysis. Here's my good news: your brain doesn't need to make rational sense. Your brain is what it is. The goal here is to tap into this energy and lifestyle that I'm calling Happy First, not to cover up your fear but to expose it. Once you turn the light on, most fears vanish. Once you learn about your true nature and real existence, there will come a day when it's difficult even to create the fear storm you used to hover beneath.

Fear can be utterly incapacitating, and it might be the only thing that stops you from carrying out a life of Happy First. Fear will prevent you from chasing down those dreams and goals. Anxiety will raise its ugly head in many, many forms to keep you small. Or, in many cases, that fear will keep you large and holding onto extra fat through behaviors that no longer serve your higher self. Fear will keep you hidden and isolated. Fear will stop you from making friends and sharing your knowledge and wisdom. Fear will prevent you from allowing your spouse to love you. Fear will stop you from teaching and learning. Fear can get so paralyzing it can stop you from leaving your home.

Many people, even when they do leave their homes, don't truly leave themselves. They don't show themselves to others. Instead, they exist in a state of perpetual terror. Happy First is a way to move past fear, past our fear of dying, living, and standing in our role as friends and parents and spouses. We step into the light of day. When your energy and drive come from a place that never stops and never changes, you can show up. For you, showing up might mean eating something other than Cheetos. It might mean getting out and taking a walk. It might mean meandering around the grocery store instead of having groceries delivered or doing curbside pickup, not because of a virus, but because you were afraid to interact.

Sometimes the fear is as stereotypical as, "What will they think of me?" Sometimes it's more insidious, like, "What will I think of myself?" Sure, we go to work and we talk to people. But many of us hide behind a facade of competence, or intimidation, or smallness. When we rely on our own limited reserves, every interaction takes something away. We get smaller and smaller and more afraid. We start to hate our jobs and blame the job, the coworkers, the boss. We get a "better" job and think the fault lies with the clients or the paycheck. We're trying to exist drinking from a small cup, when in reality, you can thrive with an infinite wellspring at your disposal.

When you learn to move past fear and see the energy available to you, you can never unsee it. You no longer need a "10 steps to a better marriage" article. You just somehow show up as a kind and loving spouse. Even weirder, you wonder when your spouse became so amazing. You each care about your days, you support each other's goals and dreams and hopes. You go to work and interact and give because you're not afraid of running out anymore.

At the end of the day, you have energy for exercise and play because you no longer need to hide from the day at the bottom of a bottle or a shopping bag. The day isn't wearing on you. The day supports you and you float. Where is the fear in that? Where is the fear of opening up? Somehow it has just gone.

The fear is still there, though. I know this; I can feel it. It's a really big world out there. That world is uncontrollable. Buildings topple, regimes topple, relationships topple. Do you think the people that decimate buildings out of acts of terror are living from a space of Happy First? The very word terrorism speaks of spreading fear. Even playground bullies want us to be afraid. It keeps us small. It keeps us obedient. Oddly, we might all become more obedient if we could live with a spirit of freedom. That's why Americans fight so hard for our liberties. Unfortunately, we often turn around and impose our own restrictions. We have all the freedom in the world, yet we live from a space so small that we cut ourselves off at the knees.

The laws cannot mandate that you live from a place of Happy First. This is an individual pursuit. You can't make your spouse or your coworker or your child live from a place of Happy First. This is all you. Only you have your fears. Only you walk your path. But by bringing more love and light and joy into the world, you create a different world. You affect your family, your community, your office, your town, and your world.

If you have fear today, that doesn't mean you have to

have it tomorrow. Your life can instantaneously change. As I discussed in chapter 19, "Doubt Is Inevitable," the fear might come back, tomorrow, or in a minute—but it doesn't have to stay. You know what to do. Use a state changer, talk to a trusted friend or mentor, read a book, listen to music. You know where to go to tap in. You know where you go to connect with that Happy First energy. The only way out of fear is to come from a different place. You can't tamp it down from the outside; that'll just make it explode later. When we stuff fear down, it just gets worse and bigger. You're not afraid of the circumstance, you're afraid of your thoughts about the circumstance. So, start changing your thoughts. Think about a flower, a song, your cat that yells during the meeting with caps lock on. Breathe.

There has yet to be a situation in your life you didn't successfully make it through. The problem is you can't handle situations that aren't there. Fear is about the monsters in your mind; it'll have different names and wear different faces, but it's all still your fear. It's not the circumstance. Walk through it. Walk past it. You've got a source of infinite energy. Use it and let it flow right through you to move you to a better thought, a better moment.

# Chapter 21
# No Need to Bounce

Although you may need to revisit your Happy First grounding thoughts multiple times a day, or an hour, that doesn't mean you have to be "resilient." That word is used pretty consistently, and for good reason. When it feels like you are buffeted by life circumstances, you must bounce back. This concept is absolutely needed. But I propose that instead of thinking life is about getting knocked down and having to stand back up, you don't look at circumstances as knocking you down. You simply stand. Events may have to be dealt with, but you stand like the palm tree. You sway in that hurricane and you stand strong. You now come from a place where your roots run deep. Your foundation is strong. You're not standing on shaky ground any longer. You don't have a need to be resilient—because now you're stable. You still have highs and lows, but the highs are higher and the lows are higher.

The more you tap into Happy First, the more it raises your vibration—how connected you are to your source energy—overall. You begin to see that it's okay to remain content or satisfied or even happy in the midst of adverse circumstances. Suffering is not a contest. Proving your misery doesn't make you a more worthy person. Undergoing and overcoming more trials and tribulations doesn't make you better than someone else. We all have our own battles to fight. Most of us fight them in isolation and no one can honestly know another's struggle or victory. Be kind. Instead of facing life as problem after problem, I propose that you live life on life's terms. See the world from the stance of infinite beauty. Look more quickly and easily at the potential outcome and benefits of a struggle rather than having to get there after a long period of depression or hopelessness. Stay focused on your internal work, guided by your deep knowing rather than by the calamity of circumstance.

By living from a Happy First energy, you're able to see through the current struggle. You're able to look above the weather and see the storm for what it is—nothing more than a set of changing circumstances. When you're grounded in the energy that is your birthright, you needn't fear the storm. You needn't be resilient because you never fell.

Some of my favorite literary works have been about being resilient and bouncing back. I do believe these concepts are extremely valuable for personal growth, so I'm not discounting the concept entirely. I'm simply proposing a shift in perspective on hardship. One of the most important characteristics of people who happily thrive and succeed is perseverance. Victors don't quit. They don't quit when they win. They don't quit when they lose.

# Chapter 22

# Keep the Channel Open

As we reach the end of the book, I'd like to tie all the concepts together. We've gone over how to reconnect—from daily practices to thought processes—and why they're so important. We've touched on why this reset is vital for us as individuals and for our society as a whole. We've acknowledged that external circumstances will seem to intrude upon your channeling of that Happy First energy.

Your first task now is to create an internal conduit. This is a metaphorical image that has helped me picture the way we live Happy First. Living Happy First means you ground yourself in that energy You allow that energy to help you make decisions and perform actions. Picture a warm light flowing from the roots of a tree up toward the sun.

Thoughts, decisions, and actions create your world. By cultivating this constant flow of energy, there may come a day when you don't need to tap in because this has become your default way of being. Your existence is grounded in that energy, that power. You have an infinite source of hope and joy and perseverance. Your job is to realize that possibility. My job is to show you it exists.

My goal is not for you to do what I say or even what I do. I don't want you to reach your goals the way I reach my goals. You'll have your own wonderfully unique path to success. I'm here to show you that there's a different way than trudging down the beaten path. I'm here to open up the thought that reality may not exactly be what you've learned. I can show you that changing your thoughts and your thought processes to align with living Happy First can be an instantaneous positive change in your world. In any way you can, the way to amplify these good feelings is going to be unique to you and even unique to the day.

The next chapter lists quick state changers to turn your reality upside down. That way, when you come to a fork in the road, you can just flip to that chapter and pick one. If worse comes to worst, you just open it up and do something. Life isn't really trial and error. Life is action and error. We don't try things. We *do* things. You have thoughts and you have actions. Your actions are what define you. Your thoughts do contribute in a way greater than we've ever realized, but they're still manifested as action. No matter the action, you'll always obtain a result. Is the result getting you closer to your real self? If not, adjust the thoughts and the actions follow.

The more authors and speakers and coaches realize this, the more we will all benefit. One person knowing the truth tells two more. Those two go on to tell their family and friends. I believe this is the only way to affect change. Laws and governments will be needed until we can emotionally and mentally evolve. But laws and governments aren't the way to make your life more fulfilling on a daily basis. Granted, driving the wrong way on the highway is likely going to make your day a lot less fulfilling and possibly truly short. The way to create the life that you feel is within your grasp is to work from a place of internal peace.

Energetic laws will play a larger role from this place. For example, when you give anger to someone, you're more than likely going to get anger back. When you give kindness to someone, you may get anger back, but often it will fizzle quickly and most times it won't even present itself. Life shows you what you show it. Screaming at the wood stove to make you warm without first putting wood in does nothing except make you miserable. When we speak and act from a place of giving and kindness, everyone wins.

Life is meant to be enjoyed. You're meant to live from a place of happiness, and that place of happiness isn't a destination. Joy isn't something you attain when you learn how to meditate for half an hour every day. You're born from energy that creates your joy, contentment, and happiness. That energy sits at the core of your being, and it never changes. The more you let go of your learned negative programs, the more of that energy shines through.

That's why I've discussed everything from your food intake to your sleep to your relationships. I discussed my annoying cat (since I wrote that chapter, he's also broken the C key on my laptop because he's heavy). I probably should have written a chapter on the rock in your shoe. One little pebble can create an epic ruckus. It's flabbergasting, the little things that can disrupt our flow. But we are human. We live in the real world. Things happen. But *we* also happen. We are each individual miracles. We don't need excess food or exercise or wine or excitement to be happy. There's nothing wrong with an occasional nonharmful indulgence. But once you discover what really sits with your moral code and realize where that comes from, it becomes remarkably simple to make decisions. Some of my examples are from friends and coworkers, some are mine. I look forward to hearing yours.

The wider that channel is open, the easier daily decisions become. Being happy isn't just about getting all the things. Being happy is about being all the things being true, being honest, being open. It's about being loving and being kind, especially to yourself. Sometimes living Happy First is also about being wrong. Choosing kind over being right doesn't come naturally to me. I want to be right. But maybe I don't know best. Admitting that I was wrong about what I did even to myself and maybe to a trusted friend or an advisor—that's honesty. The more honest you get, the more open that channel stays.

I need to make sure one thing is unequivocally stated. I do not believe happiness requires anything. Sure, as Michael Neill told us, it's OK to want both peace and a nice piece of real estate, but happiness comes from inside. External circumstances can enhance our life, but attainment of them does not make you happy. You are indeed Happy First.

Keep reading and take a look at the next chapter, where I provide a simple list of actions that can help you get or keep the channel open. These are things that may connect you to nature, connect you to yourself, or connect you to other people. Life is all about connection. You're not out here alone, so there's no need to pretend you are any longer. Even today, you've connected with me.

# Chapter 23

# Simple Practices

Some easy ways to tap into that Happy First energy:

1. Being outside
2. Gardening
3. Cooking
4. Meditating
5. Listening to music
6. Swimming
7. Writing poetry
8. Walking
9. Petting your pet
10. Brushing your hair
11. Making cookies
12. Lifting weights
13. Calling a friend
14. Texting a colleague
15. Having a picnic
16. Reading a novel

17. Looking at the stars
18. Riding your bike
19. Having sex
20. Taking a class
21. Making pottery
22. Going for a run
23. Calling your family
24. Doing pushups
25. Eating a cookie
26. Painting
27. Listening to a podcast
28. Smiling
29. Going to a playground
30. Reading a biography
31. Praying
32. Exploring colors
33. Going shopping
34. Doing yoga
35. Floating in the pool
36. Sitting in the grass
37. Looking at flowers
38. Going to church
39. Drinking ice cold water on a hot day

40. Lighting a favorite candle
41. Walking your dog on their agenda
42. Looking at the clouds
43. Going to bed early
44. Getting your things ready the night before
45. Reading a magazine
46. Writing a letter
47. Sitting on a park bench
48. Going for a hike
49. Doodling
50. Asking questions
51. _____ (Do what feels right to you!)

# Chapter 24

# Nowhere to Go

The simple practices, or state changers, in chapter 23 might look like 50 simple practices to get you where you want to be. Instead, it's the beginning of a list of infinite actions to get you in touch with who you *are*. Remember, there's nowhere to go. You're already there. The whole premise behind Happy First is that you don't have to be something else to attain your goals. You're at a perfect starting point just as you are. You are that energy, light, and love that equals happiness. You are that kind response to your screaming child. You are that loving hug that you gave to your spouse. Because your knowing comes from that deep, deep intelligence that was there before anything, you have no need to fear.

Instead of hiding, you can live. Maybe for the first time in your life, you can live. You can wake up in the morning and be good with who you are—your body, your attitude, your energy level. And at the end of the day, you can be satisfied with the tasks you accomplished, the interactions you had, and the person you were. No longer do you need to spend your days setting goals of being kinder or gentler. You're already more loving. Start with yourself. Knowing that an everlasting source of energy is there for the taking—infinite and abundant, not exclusive—is all you need to know and practice.

As we talked about in part 1, sure, you can set goals. Maybe you want to finish college, or start. Maybe you want to do an Ironman or learn to run. Maybe you want to learn to sew or paint or write poetry. Most things are simply skills you don't have. Yes, you must invest energy to gain knowledge or strength. But no longer do you have to live in fear that you may not complete your task. That fear is manufactured and unnecessary. If you want to do something, do it. It's often said that if you wish to be a writer, write. You are as you identify yourself.

Remind yourself every morning and every night that words matter. The words you say and the words you use define your life. No longer can you blame your perceived lack of success on the fact that you don't have the energy. You *are* the energy. No longer can you blame your slow progress on the fact that there isn't enough money. You know now that everything is present in abundance. There is plenty of thriving to be had. If you forget, pause, and remember. Put that energy at the center of your day. Some of us don't know what it's like to not live in fear. Fear of failure, fear of success, fear of abandonment, fear of not being abandoned, fear of trying, fear of not trying. You name it, we've all felt it.

You do not have to live there. You aren't that. You are, in fact, what you say you are. You come from that infinite source energy.

When the thought tornado strikes, stand in your calm. You are the voice of reason. The voice of reason is the voice of truth. Truth comes from something that's older than you and smarter than you and more loving than you. Your goal is to be a channel for that energy. The less you resist it, the more it flows. And the more you resist it, the hotter and more uncomfortable it gets. That's why we eat and drink and smoke and escape. We feel compelled to cover up the heat. We "need" to cover up the discomfort.

Instead, I want you to peel off that discomfort, layer by layer, to uncover your true nature. Or just rip off the Band-Aid. Do what feels right to you. Happiness is there for the taking. This process doesn't have to be long and grueling. The physical effects may take some time, but changing your perspective is instantaneous. I ask you as we finish up our time together here to entertain the notion that you can live Happy First—starting … right … now.

# Acknowledgments

I would like to thank the following people for helping me both with this writing and with the experiences that brought me to the knowledge of Happy First. There are so many others who have affected my life not mentioned—not out of lack of gratitude, but for lack of space. You are all in my mind and heart.

Thank you to Barb Rollins for her unwavering support in my recovery and writing processes. She has so much to give as a mentor and author. Thank you to Patti Cooper for constantly reminding me that there is a different way.

Thank you to my dad, Marty, for enduring brainstorming sessions *ad nauseum* and often playing devil's advocate. I can't thank you enough. Thanks to my mom, Sandy, for teaching me so many things that became springboards in both life and this book.

Thank you to my longstanding friends Suzie and Erin; you're always there even when it's too much time since we've spoken. The same goes for my cousin Danielle, who is always more like a sibling than a cousin.

Thanks to my grandma Joan, who showed me that even at 88 years old, your life could take on new meaning and have a new beauty to it. Thank you to my grandpa Jim, who guides me as a person and a doctor both in life and death.

Thank you to Matthew, our son, who listens to me rattle on about things his little brain does not yet understand. He's heard lots of book concepts so far!

Thank you to Courtney, Brandi, Cindy, Hailey, and Meghan. You have walked (and run) with me time and time again, in peace and craziness. Thank you for being my tribe.

Thank you to the friends I've made at work. I've had so many teachers there and in training that there are too many to mention. But I really appreciate Eva, Afton, Brett, Neil, Kaetlyn, and Chris for an unbelievable number of life-changing conversations and experiences.

Thank you to Tracy Sanson for introducing me to the fact that I can always add "or better." Thank you to Jill, my SPS accountability buddy, for blazing a clear-cut trail, and to Chandler Bolt for creating a system to begin making my dreams into reality. Thank you to Sloane Kini for connecting with me on our very first coaching call and making me believe that dreams are happening.

Last but never least, thank you to my husband, Greg, for being my biggest teacher of all, my biggest supporter, and my strongest anchor in this storm of life.

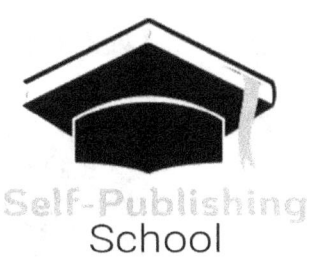
Self-Publishing School

# Now It's Your Turn

Discover the EXACT three-step blueprint you need to become a bestselling author in as little as three months.

Self-Publishing School helped me, and now I want them to help you with this FREE resource to begin outlining your book!

Even if you're busy, bad at writing, or don't know where to start, you CAN write a bestseller and build your best life.

With tools and experience across a variety of niches and professions, Self-Publishing School is a great resource to take your book to the finish line!

DON'T WAIT

Say "YES" to becoming a bestseller:

https://self-publishingschool.com/friend/


Follow the steps on the page to get a FREE resource to get started on your book and unlock a discount to get started with Self-Publishing School.

# Would You Help?

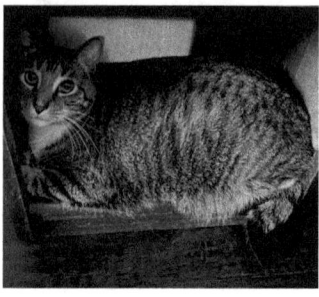

Bennie the caps-loving cat ♥

**Thank you for reading my book!**

I really appreciate all your feedback, and I love hearing what you have to say. I need your input to make the next version of this book and my future books better.

Please leave me an honest review on Amazon letting me know what you thought of the book.

Thanks so much!

*Moe*

CPSIA information can be obtained
at www.ICGtesting.com
Printed in the USA
LVHW081048100221
678920LV00025B/624/J